Sensei Self Development

Mental Health Chronicles Series

Practicing Self-Compassion

Sensei Paul David

Copyright Page

Sensei Self Development -
Practicing Self-Compassion,
by Sensei Paul David

Copyright © 2023

All rights reserved.

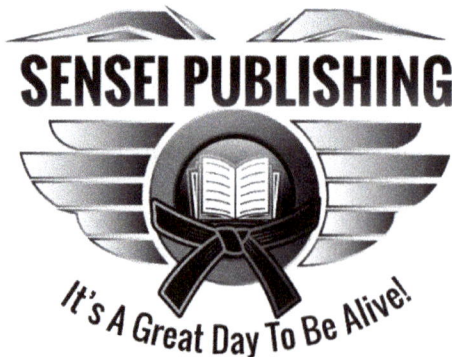

SENSEI PUBLISHING

It's A Great Day To Be Alive!

www.senseipublishing.com

@senseipublishing
#senseipublishing

Get/Share Your FREE SSD Mental Health Chronicles at

www.senseiselfdevelopment.care

or

CLICK HERE

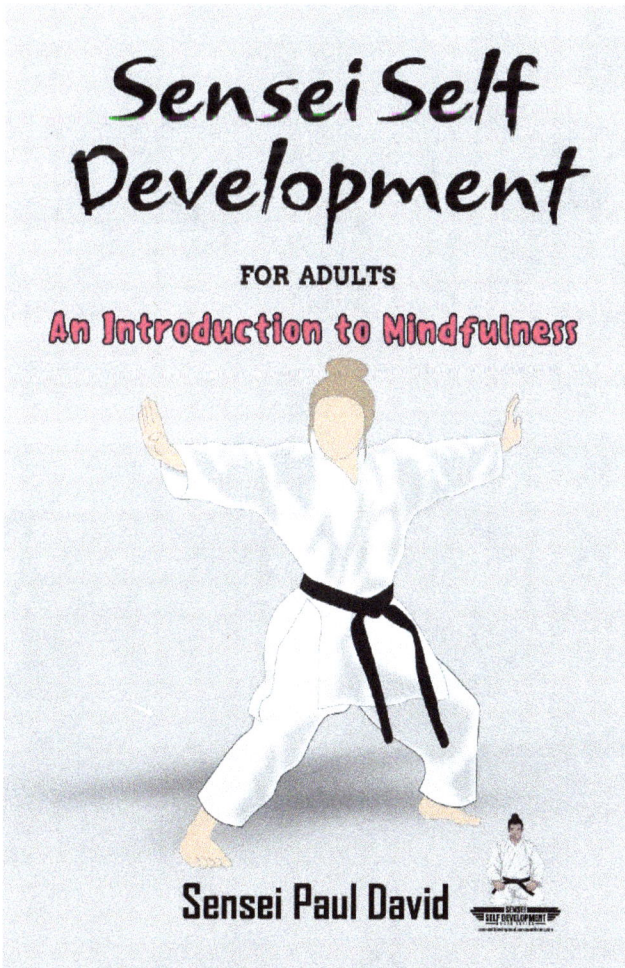

Check Out The SSD Chronicles Series CLICK HERE

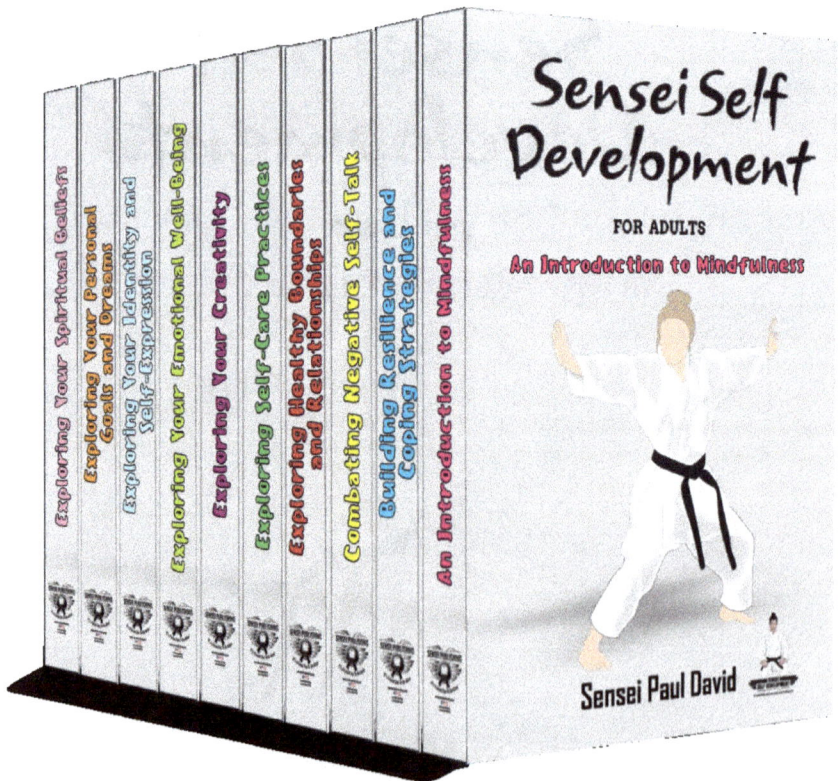

Exploring Your Spiritual Beliefs

Exploring Your Personal Goals and Dreams

Exploring Your Identity and Self-Expression

Exploring Your Emotional Well-Being

Exploring Your Creativity

Exploring Self-Care Practices

Exploring Healthy Boundaries and Relationships

Combating Negative Self-Talk

Building Resilience and Coping Strategies

An Introduction to Mindfulness

Sensei Self Development

FOR ADULTS

An Introduction to Mindfulness

Sensei Paul David

Dedication

To those who courageously take action towards self-improvement - you are helping to evolve the world for generations to come.

- It's a great day to be alive!

If Found Please Contact:

_____

Reward If Found:

_____

MY
COMMITMENT

I, _____

commit to writing This Sensei Self
Development Journal for at least 10 days in a
row, starting: _____

Writing this journal is valuable to me because:

_____

_____

_____

_____

_____

_____

If I finish a minimum of 10 consecutive days of
writing in this journal, I will reward myself by:

_____

_____

_____

_____

_____

_____

If I don't finish 10 days of writing this journal, I
will promise to:

_____

_____

_____

_____

_____

_____

I will do the following things to ensure that I
write in my Sensei Self Development Journal
every day:

_____

_____

_____

_____

_____

_____

Get/Share Your FREE All-Ages Mental Health eBook Now at

www.senseiselfdevelopment.com

Or CLICK HERE

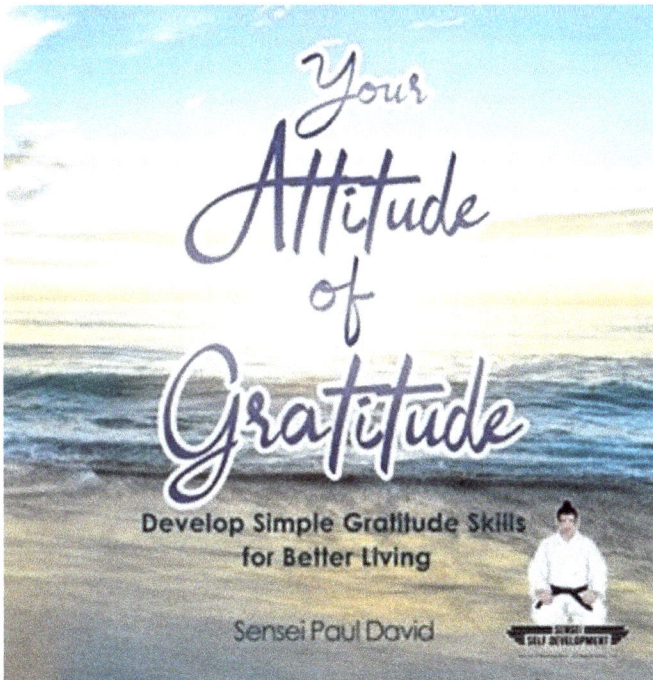

senseiselfdevelopment.com

Check Out Another Book In The
SSD BOOK SERIES:

senseipublishing.com/SSD_SERIES

CLICK HERE

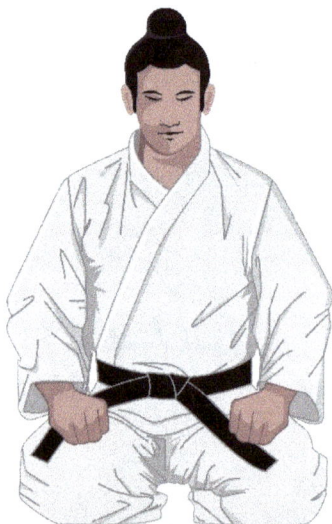

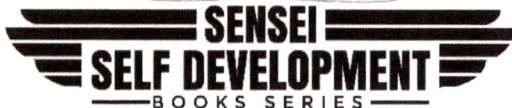

SENSEI
SELF DEVELOPMENT
BOOKS SERIES
senseiselfdevelopment.senseipublishing.com

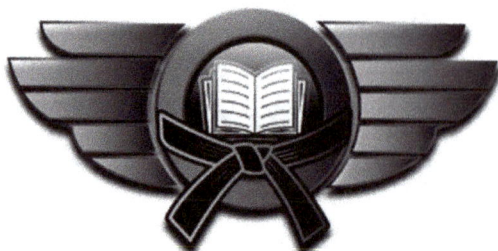

Join Our Publishing Journey!

If you would like to receive FUTURE FREE BOOKS and get to know us better, please click www.senseipublishing.com and join our newsletter by entering your email address in the pop-up box.

Follow Our Blog: senseipauldavid.ca

Follow/Like/Subscribe: Facebook, Instagram, YouTube: @senseipublishing

Scan the QR Code with your phone or tablet

to follow us on social media: Like / Subscribe / Follow

A Message From The Author:
Sensei Paul David

Dear Reader,

Welcome to the world of mental health journaling – a sacred space for self-reflection, growth, and healing. Within these pages, you hold the power to uplift your spirit, invigorate your mind, and nourish your goals.

In a world that often moves at blink-and-you'll-miss-it speed, it's crucial to make time for self-care and self-discovery.

Anxiety, stress, and emotional turbulence may have clouded your mind, making it difficult to find clarity and peace within. But fear not! Together, we will navigate the labyrinth of emotions, and experiences, helping to simplify the path to mental well-being.

This journal is not merely a bunch of blank pages awaiting your words. It is your compassionate companion, offering solace and understanding during your unique journey. Here, you are free to unburden yourself, celebrate small and large victories, and confront the challenges that may still linger.

Within the sheltered realm of these pages, there is no judgment, no expectation, and no pressure. Your unique experience and perspective hold immeasurable worth, and your voice deserves to be heard. Whether you choose to fill the lines with eloquence or simply scribble fragments of your thoughts, please remember each entry is a valuable contribution to your growth.

In this sacred space, you are challenged to take off the mask we so often wear in the outside world. It is here that you can be raw, vulnerable, and authentic – allowing your true self to be seen and embraced without reservation. By giving yourself permission to explore the depths of your emotions and confront the shadows that may lurk within, you will discover profound insights and find the healing you seek over time.

As you embark on this journaling journey, I encourage you to embrace the process itself rather than fixate solely on the outcome. Remember, it is not about reaching a certain destination or ticking off boxes on a list of accomplishments. Rather, it is about cultivating self-awareness, fostering self-compassion, and nurturing a sense of curiosity about the intricate workings of your intelligently beautiful mind.

In the quiet moments of reflection, let your pen become a bridge between your inner world and the possibilities that lie ahead. Create a sanctuary for your thoughts, fears, triumphs, and dreams. As you pour your heart onto these pages, allow your words to be a living testament to courage, resilience, and an unwavering commitment to your own well-being.

I am honored to be a part of your journey, and I believe in your ability to navigate the twists and turns with grace and resilience. Remember, you are not alone in this – countless others have walked similar paths, faced similar challenges, and emerged stronger and wiser on the other side. You have the power to reclaim all of your untapped joy, cultivate a positive mindset that serves you, and foster a deep sense of self-love and peaceful confident. – And it will take a worth effort and time.

So, open the first page of this journal with hope, curiosity, and an open heart and open mind. Embrace the transformative power of self-reflection, and allow it to guide you towards a life of greater fulfilment and peace. Each journaling session is an opportunity to not only connect with yourself but also to rekindle the light within that sometimes flickers but never extinguishes.

Remember, the pages you are about to fill are not just a record of your journey but also a testament to your strength, resilience, and indomitable spirit. Cherish this space, invest in yourself, and lct your words be an ode to the magnificent journey of becoming whole.

With great respect for your decision to evolve,

Paul

MY CONVICTION

Please circle your answers below

I am DECIDING to be patient with myself and this PROCESS each time I journal toward my improved state of mental well-being

YES   NO

"The present moment is filled with joy and happiness. If you are attentive, you will see it."

Thich Nhat Hanh

Introduction

Self-compassion is a gentle and understanding approach towards oneself, especially in moments of difficulty or failure. It's about treating yourself with the same kindness and care that you would offer to a good friend. It's a nurturing attitude, recognizing that everyone has moments of suffering or makes mistakes, and treating oneself with the same warmth and care one would offer a close friend in similar situations.

This concept hinges on the realization that imperfection and struggle are universal aspects of the human experience. When we practice self-compassion, we acknowledge our feelings and experiences without harsh judgment or self-criticism. It's about observing our own vulnerabilities with empathy and patience, rather than with negativity or harsh self-scrutiny.

The practice of self-compassion involves a balanced and mindful acknowledgment of our emotions. It encourages us to accept and understand our feelings, but also to not become overwhelmed by them. This balance helps in not over-identifying with our shortcomings or difficult emotions, enabling a more objective and kind perspective towards ourselves.

Engaging in self-compassion is fundamentally different from self-indulgence or self-pity. It's not about ignoring our faults or avoiding responsibility for our actions. Instead, it's a supportive and constructive way to confront our own failings and challenges, promoting personal growth and emotional healing.

By adopting a self-compassionate attitude, we open the door to greater self-acceptance and emotional resilience. It allows us to navigate through life's challenges with a sense of understanding and kindness towards ourselves, fostering an inner environment where growth, healing, and acceptance can flourish. Self-compassion, thus, becomes a powerful tool in building a healthier, more positive relationship with ourselves.

Studies have shown that self-compassion stands as a robust source of coping and resilience, significantly enhancing our mental and physical health. It inspires us to pursue changes and achieve our goals, not from a place of feeling inadequate, but from a place of genuine care and a desire for happiness.

Key Practices of self-compassion:

1. Self-Kindness: At the core of self-kindness is the practice of treating oneself with care and understanding rather than harsh criticism. It involves actively soothing and comforting oneself in times of distress. This might look like speaking to oneself in a gentle, encouraging voice, or acknowledging that it's okay to be imperfect. Practicing self-kindness means recognizing that suffering and feelings of inadequacy are experiences that all humans share, and responding to these feelings with sympathy and patience, rather than contempt or self-disparagement. It's about allowing oneself to be human, to make mistakes, and to learn from them without self-flagellation.

2. Common Humanity: This component involves recognizing that suffering and personal inadequacy are part of the shared human experience. It's a shift from the perspective of "I'm the only one suffering" or "I'm the only one who makes mistakes" to a more inclusive understanding that all humans struggle, and that these experiences connect us with others. Common humanity counteracts the feelings of loneliness and isolation that often accompany pain and failure. By understanding that suffering is a part of life for everyone, we develop a more compassionate and less judgmental attitude towards ourselves and others. This recognition fosters a sense of connectedness and belonging, helping to alleviate the sense of isolation that often compounds personal suffering.

3. Mindfulness: Mindfulness in the context of self-compassion involves a balanced approach to negative emotions so that feelings are neither suppressed nor exaggerated. This balanced awareness entails acknowledging and observing our painful thoughts and feelings

with openness and clarity, without attachment or over-identification. Mindfulness allows us to not be "swept away" by the intensity of our emotions, but instead to observe them as they are. This awareness creates a space where one can approach their feelings and experiences with curiosity and openness, rather than judgment and denial. It's about facing and accepting reality as it is in the present moment, which is essential for emotional healing and growth.

Each of these three components plays a crucial role in cultivating a compassionate attitude towards oneself.

Benefits of Self-Compassion

According to Dr Kristin Neff, who is a leading expert in self-compassion in the world, people who are compassionate to themselves are much less likely to be depressed, anxious and stressed and are much more likely to be happy, resilient and optimistic about their future. In short, they have better mental health.

This is not mere speculation. It is measurable. The concept of self-compassion holds a tangible and significant power that goes beyond just thoughts and feelings; it actually manifests in our physical bodies. When we engage in self-soothing, we activate the mammalian care-giving system. A key aspect of this system is the release of oxytocin, a hormone that enhances feelings of trust, calm, safety, generosity, and connectedness, and it plays a crucial role in fostering warmth and compassion towards ourselves. Oxytocin is naturally released in various social interactions, such as during breastfeeding, parent-child bonding, or even through gentle physical touch. This suggests that self-compassion can be a powerful catalyst for oxytocin release, given that our bodies respond similarly to emotions directed towards ourselves as they do to those directed towards others.

On the other hand, self-criticism activates a very different bodily response. The amygdala, an ancient part of our brain, is designed to quickly detect threats. When faced with a threat, it triggers the fight-or-flight response, increasing blood pressure, adrenaline, and cortisol. This system, originally meant for physical threats, also responds to emotional threats, whether from others or self-imposed. Intriguingly, research shows that fostering feelings of self-compassion can actually lower cortisol levels, the stress hormone.

In one study, participants were guided to imagine receiving and feeling compassion deeply. They were prompted with phrases encouraging them to feel enveloped by compassion and loving-kindness. Those who followed these instructions showed lower cortisol levels compared to a control group, along with increased heart rate variability. This suggests that a sense of safety and openness, reflected in heart rate variability, can be enhanced through self-compassion. Essentially, by offering compassion to themselves, participants' hearts responded by becoming more open and less defensive.

Thus, when we address our painful feelings with self-compassion, we're not only altering our mental and emotional state but also positively influencing our body chemistry. It's a testament to the profound impact of self-compassion, intertwining our emotional well-being with our physical health.

To summarize, self-compassion will reduce your anxiety and make you feel warm. And you will enjoy all the health benefits that come associated with superior mental health.

What Self-Compassion Is Not?

Self-compassion vs. Self-pity

Self-compassion, as opposed to self-pity, is a nurturing and expansive way to approach our own challenges. When we fall into self-pity, we can become engulfed in our own problems, losing sight of the fact that everyone faces difficulties. Self-pity often leads us to feel uniquely burdened and disconnected from others, intensifying a sense of solitude in our suffering.

In contrast, self-compassion opens our hearts to a shared human experience. It reminds us that we are not alone in our struggles; others have walked similar paths. With self-compassion, we recognize our challenges as part of the broader human experience, enabling us to feel more connected and less alone.

Moreover, self-pity can trap us in our own emotional turmoil, making it hard to see beyond our immediate situation. We might become consumed by our feelings, losing the ability to step back and view our circumstances with a more balanced and objective lens. Self-compassion, however, offers us this "mental space." It's like stepping back and viewing our situation through the eyes of a compassionate friend. This shift allows us to see our experiences in a broader context - recognizing that it's normal and natural for human beings to encounter hardships. This broader perspective brings not only comfort but also a sense of groundedness in the midst of our trials.

Self-compassion is not Self Indulgence

Some people criticise self-compassion, fearing it might lead to self-indulgent behavior. They worry that under the guise of being kind to themselves, they might end up justifying unhelpful actions - like spending a whole day watching TV to alleviate stress, which is actually an act of self-indulgence rather than genuine self-compassion.

True self-compassion is about seeking long-term happiness and health, not just short-term pleasure. It involves making choices that are truly beneficial for oneself, even if they might be uncomfortable in the moment. For example, choosing to exercise, save money, or quit smoking might not provide immediate gratification, but these actions lead to greater health and lasting happiness. They are acts of self-compassion because they demonstrate care for one's future well-being, as opposed to self-indulgence, which often focuses on fleeting pleasures that may ultimately be detrimental.

Furthermore, self-compassion offers a nurturing alternative to the self-flagellation approach. Often, people try to motivate themselves with criticism and shame, thinking that being hard on themselves will spur change. However, this method can backfire, as the fear of self-hatred might prevent someone from facing difficult truths about themselves. In contrast, self-compassion provides a safe and supportive space for personal growth and self-awareness. It allows individuals to acknowledge their weaknesses and challenges without fear of self-condemnation, fostering a kind and understanding environment for change. The care and motivation inherent in self-compassion become powerful forces for growth, encouraging us to see ourselves clearly and kindly, and to make changes that are in our best interest.

Self-Compassion is not Self-Esteem or Self-Confidence

Self-compassion and self-esteem, while related, serve distinct roles in how we perceive and treat ourselves. Self-compassion isn't about inflating our ego or self-worth as self-esteem often is; rather, it's about a balanced and kind acknowledgment of our imperfections and limitations. It allows us to view ourselves from a realistic standpoint, embracing both our strengths and weaknesses.

In many aspects of modern culture, there's an emphasis on projecting confidence, sometimes even to the point of delusion. This approach can be risky, as feigning confidence might lead us to overestimate our abilities, a situation that can have negative outcomes. This is where self-compassion offers a grounding alternative. Unlike the potentially misleading nature of overconfidence, self-compassion encourages us to accept ourselves as we are, flaws and all.

Self-compassion is about treating ourselves with kindness and understanding, akin to how we would treat a loved one. It recognizes that being human involves imperfections and struggles, and accepts these as part of the shared human experience. This approach helps to maintain a realistic view of ourselves, without exaggerating our strengths or weaknesses.

Self-confidence encourages us to squash any revolting thought that appears in our mind. This can lead to a mental discomfort as one tries to rein in these doubts and insecurities. On the contrary, self-compassion does not try to quell any legitimate criticism. It encourages us to say, "of course I have problems. I am only human."

In a study featured in the Journal of Personality and Social Psychology, participants were asked to make a video describing themselves, aware that they'd be evaluated on traits like likability and intelligence. The findings were intriguing: individuals with a strong sense of self-compassion maintained a steady emotional state, regardless of how they were rated. However, those with high self-esteem didn't take neutral feedback well. They got upset and blamed external reasons for not receiving exceptional ratings.

Have Self-Compassion for Your Inner Critic

We all know the sting of harsh self-criticism – those moments when we berate ourselves with thoughts like "I'm an idiot!" or "No one will ever love me." But why do we engage in this painful self-talk? Often, when we question this habit, we end up layering even more criticism onto ourselves.

It's important to realize that self-criticism, though harsh and unhelpful, is an attempt by our inner critic to protect us. It's a misguided effort to keep us safe, rooted in our basic human survival systems. We have evolved with a threat defense system, where the amygdala plays a key role in activating fight, flight, freeze, or submit responses. These responses can be life-saving in the wild, but in our complex human lives, they often backfire, especially when the threat is to our self-concept rather than physical safety.

This system might manifest as emotional self-attack (fight), anxiety and restlessness (flight), rumination (freeze), or accepting negative self-judgments (submit). Engaging in these strategies increases stress, as our body floods with adrenaline and cortisol, and it's particularly taxing because we are both the attacker and the victim. This chronic stress can lead to long-term emotional and physical health issues.

However, it's crucial to recognize that our inner critic isn't our enemy. It's trying to protect us, albeit in a counterproductive way. Marshall

Rosenberg, known for his work in Non-Violent Communication, views self-criticism as a "tragic expression of an unmet need." It's an expression of care that unfortunately makes us feel worse and doesn't motivate us effectively. For instance, calling yourself a "lazy slob" for not going to the gym is your inner critic's way of showing concern for your health and social acceptance, albeit in a misguided manner.

Fortunately, we have another system at our disposal: the attachment/affiliation system, integral to our evolution as mammals. This system responds to warmth and affection, calming us down and promoting emotional safety. It's the system that soothes us, reducing cortisol levels and activating the parasympathetic nervous system.

So, the next time you catch yourself amid self-criticism, instead of getting caught in a loop of criticism, try acknowledging your inner critic's intent and then offer yourself-compassion. This approach is not only more effective in reducing stress and anxiety, but it also creates a space for emotional balance and wiser decision-making. Giving yourself-compassion moves you out of the threat defense mode and into a more nurturing, caring state. It's a kinder, more effective way to address your needs and challenges.

How to Practise self-compassion

1. Treat Yourself Like a Friend

Imagine you've just had a particularly challenging day at work, where nothing seemed to go right. You missed a deadline, and your boss expressed disappointment in your performance. Feeling deflated, you start berating yourself: "I can't do anything right," "I'm such a failure." This is a crucial moment to practice self-compassion.

In this moment, instead of sinking into self-criticism, pause and consider how you would respond if a close friend were in your situation. Would you berate them as you're doing to yourself? Most likely, you'd offer words of comfort and encouragement. Try to extend this same kindness to yourself. Speak to yourself in a gentle, understanding tone. Remind yourself that everyone faces setbacks and that one bad day doesn't define your entire worth or ability.

Use this scenario as an opportunity to reframe your thoughts. Replace "I'm a failure" with "I'm learning and growing." Acknowledge your feelings of disappointment or frustration, but also remind yourself that these are temporary and part of the human experience. Be as compassionate to yourself as you would be to a friend in a similar situation.

Here is an exercise you can try:

1. Reflect on Supporting a Friend:
   - Recall a time when a friend was struggling or feeling bad about themselves.
   - Write down your actions, the comforting words you used, and the tone of your voice.

2. Self-Reflection:
   - Think about a time when you felt bad about yourself or faced a challenge.

- Note your reactions, the things you said to yourself, and your tone.

3. Notice the Difference:

- Compare your responses in both situations.
- Reflect on any differences in how you treat a friend vs. how you treat yourself.

4. Understanding the Discrepancy:

- Contemplate why these differences exist.
- Identify any fears or beliefs that influence your self-response.

5. Imagine a Shift:

- Envision responding to your own struggles with the same kindness you show a friend.
- Consider how this change in approach could impact your emotional well-being and resilience.

2. Mindfulness, Common Humanity, and Self-kindness

Remember in the beginning we talked about three key practices of self-compassion. Here is a step by step approach you can take to implement them.

Step 1: Mindfulness: Catch Your Thoughts and Feelings.

Our inner thoughts can often feel like a relentless buzz in the background. A helpful approach to managing this internal chatter is to listen to these thoughts with patience and understanding.

The next time you find yourself slipping up, take a moment to notice the critical things you say to yourself. For instance:

- After accidentally spilling something, you might reprimand yourself, "I am so clumsy"

- After submitting a project, you might tell yourself, "That work wasn't good enough."

- Following a comment in a meeting, you might reflect, "That comment I made was so unnecessary."

Paying attention to these thoughts as they arise allows you to recognize them for what they are: irrationally critical or negative thoughts. When you catch yourself getting caught up in this spiral of criticism, pause and gently remind yourself, "That's a very critical thought."

This may seem like a small action, but it is a crucial first step. Recognizing and acknowledging these critical thoughts is essential in starting to change them. It's about understanding and gradually shifting how you speak to yourself, laying the groundwork for a more compassionate internal dialogue.

Step 2: Common Humanity: Embracing Our Shared Experience

When you encounter hardships or negative emotions, it's essential to remember the concept of common humanity. This idea centers on the understanding that you are not alone in your experiences. Challenges, pain, and feelings of inadequacy are universal aspects of the human condition that everyone faces at some point. By embracing common humanity, you acknowledge that your struggles are part of a larger, shared human experience. Here's how you can delve deeper into this understanding:

1. Acknowledge Shared Feelings:

   - Remind yourself that what you're feeling isn't unique to you. Others have felt this way too. Say to yourself, "Other people feel this way."

2. Recognize You're Not Alone:

   - In moments of difficulty, it's easy to feel isolated. Counter this by reminding yourself, "I'm not alone." This helps to diminish the loneliness that often accompanies suffering.

3. Understand the Universality of Struggle:

   - Reflect on the fact that all humans face trials and tribulations. Reinforce this by telling yourself, "We all struggle in our lives." This perspective can bring comfort and a sense of connection to others.

By focusing on common humanity, you foster a sense of belonging and connectedness. This realization can be incredibly comforting and reduce feelings of isolation and alienation. It's a reminder that everyone goes through tough times and that experiencing difficulties doesn't make you any less competent or worthy. Embracing our shared humanity is a crucial step in practicing self-compassion and developing a kinder, more understanding relationship with yourself.

Step 3: Self-Kindness

This step involves directly addressing yourself with kindness and compassion. Ask yourself, "What do I need to hear right now to express kindness to myself?" Choose a phrase or statement that resonates with your current situation, something that provides comfort and encouragement. Here are some examples:

- "May I give myself the compassion that I need."

- "May I learn to accept myself as I am."
- "May I forgive myself for my mistakes."
- "May I find strength in this challenge."
- "May I be patient with my progress."

You can use this practice at any time, whether day or night. It's a powerful way to remind yourself of the three aspects of self-compassion—mindfulness, common humanity, and self-kindness—especially in moments when you need them the most. By regularly practicing this, you reinforce a compassionate and caring approach towards yourself, enhancing your resilience and well-being.

Self-Compassion Journal

Consider starting a self-compassion journal for a week or more. Journaling can be a powerful tool for emotional expression, enhancing both mental and physical wellness. In the evening, find a quiet moment to reflect on the day. In your journal, note any moments you felt bad about, judged yourself for, or experienced pain.

Mindfulness:

Focus on the emotions that surfaced from self-judgment or challenging situations. Write about your feelings - sadness, shame, fear, stress - with acceptance and without exaggeration. For example, "I felt frustrated and reacted harshly, which made me feel foolish afterward."

Common Humanity:

Connect your experiences to the broader human experience. Acknowledge that imperfection is part of being human and that everyone has painful experiences. For instance, "Everyone overreacts sometimes. My reaction was influenced by being late and the traffic situation."

Self-Kindness:

Offer yourself kind, comforting words. Reassure yourself with understanding and gentle self-talk. For example, "It's okay, everyone has moments of frustration. I understand why you reacted that way. Let's try to show extra patience and kindness moving forward."

Regularly practicing these three aspects of self-compassion in your journaling can help structure your thoughts and solidify them in your memory. As you continue this practice, you'll find it increasingly influencing your daily life, strengthening your self-compassion.

Providing a Supportive Touch

Supportive touch is a simple and effective way to comfort yourself when you're feeling down. It activates the care system and the parasympathetic nervous system, helping you calm down and feel safe. While it might initially feel awkward, your body naturally responds to this gesture of warmth and care. Physical touch is known to release oxytocin, create a sense of security, soothe emotional distress, and reduce cardiovascular stress.

To practice this, try placing your hand on your heart or another comforting spot on your body during difficult times. Do this several times a day for at least a week and observe how it impacts your mood and stress levels. This method taps into our body's innate ability to self-soothe.

If placing a hand over your heart feels uncomfortable, it's perfectly okay to find an alternative soothing touch that works for you. Everyone has different areas where a gentle touch can feel reassuring. Here are some options you might want to explore:

- Resting one hand gently on your cheek.
- Cradling your face softly in your hands.
- Gently stroking your arms.
- Crossing your arms and giving yourself a gentle squeeze.
- Rubbing your chest gently, perhaps in circular motions.
- Placing a hand on your abdomen.
- Trying one hand on your abdomen and the other over your heart.
- Cupping one hand in the other and resting them in your lap.

Feel free to experiment with these different touches to discover which one provides the most comfort and reassurance for you.

Date ___ / ___ / ___: S   M   T   W   Th   F   S

I feel:
(please circle)

because _____   because _____   because _____   because _____   because _____
_____   _____   _____   _____   _____

Today I Am Grateful For
1. _____
2. _____
3. _____

What could help transform today into a remarkable day?

Reflective Writing

How have my experiences with self-compassion impacted my view of myself?

_____

_____

_____

_____

_____

_____

_____

_____

What is self-compassion?

a. Showing kindness and understanding towards oneself
b. Being critical and judgmental towards oneself
c. Ignoring one's own needs and feelings
d. Comparing oneself to others and feeling inadequate

Answer: a. Showing kindness and understanding towards oneself

Date ___ / ___ / ___ : S   M   T   W   Th   F   S

I feel:
(please circle)

because   because   because   because   because
_____ _____ _____ _____ _____
_____ _____ _____ _____ _____

Today I Am Grateful For

1. _____
2. _____
3. _____

What could help transform today into a remarkable day?

Reflective Writing

What do I believe is the most important aspect of self-compassion?

_____

_____

_____

_____

_____

_____

_____

_____

Which of the following is an example of practicing self-compassion?

a. Berating yourself for making a mistake
b. Ignoring your emotions and pushing through difficult situations
c. Taking a break and engaging in self-care when feeling overwhelmed
d. Comparing your achievements to others and feeling inadequate

Answer: c. Taking a break and engaging in self-care when feeling overwhelmed

Date ___ / ___ / ___ : S   M   T   W   Th   F   S

I feel:
(please circle)

because   because   because   because   because

_____ _____ _____ _____ _____

_____ _____ _____ _____ _____

Today I Am Grateful For

1. _____
2. _____
3. _____

What could help transform today into a remarkable day?

Reflective Writing

What have I learned about myself through
practicing self-compassion?

_____

_____

_____

_____

_____

_____

_____

Why is self-compassion important?

a. It helps build strong interpersonal relationships
b. It promotes feelings of self-worth and acceptance
c. It reduces stress and anxiety levels
d. All of the above

All Are Correct - Choose The Response You Feel Is Most Important To Remember

Date ___ / ___ / ___ : S   M   T   W   Th   F   S

I feel:
(please circle)

because   because   because   because   because
_____   _____   _____   _____   _____
_____   _____   _____   _____   _____

Today I Am Grateful For
1. _____
2. _____
3. _____

What could help transform today into a remarkable day?

Reflective Writing
How has my self-compassion practice changed my relationship with myself?

_____

_____

_____

_____

_____

_____

_____

Which of the following is a component of self-compassion?

a. Self-judgment
b. Self-criticism
c. Self-acceptance
d. Self-acceptance

Answer: d. Self-acceptance

Date ___ / ___ / ___: S M T W Th F S

I feel:
(please circle)

because _____ _____
because _____ _____
because _____ _____
because _____ _____
because _____ _____

Today I Am Grateful For

1. _____
2. _____
3. _____

What could help transform today into a remarkable day?

Reflective Writing

What are the most difficult aspects of self-compassion?

_____

_____

_____

_____

_____

_____

_____

Which statement best describes self-compassion?

a. It is only for individuals facing major life challenges.
b. It is a sign of weakness.
c. It is a valuable tool for navigating life's ups and downs.
d. It can only be practiced by highly self-confident individuals.

Answer: c. It is a valuable tool for navigating life's ups and downs.

Date ___ / ___ / ___ : S   M   T   W   Th   F   S

I feel:
(please circle)

because   because   because   because   because
_____ _____ _____ _____ _____
_____ _____ _____ _____ _____

Today I Am Grateful For

1. _____
2. _____
3. _____

What could help transform today into a remarkable day?

Reflective Writing

How do I use self-compassion to navigate my emotions?

_____

_____

_____

_____

_____

_____

_____

Which action demonstrates self-compassion?

a. Constantly comparing oneself to others
b. Setting unrealistic expectations and berating oneself for not meeting them
c. Offering oneself kindness and understanding during difficult times
d. Ignoring one's own needs and prioritizing others at all times

Answer: c. Offering oneself kindness and understanding during difficult times

Date ___/___/___: S M T W Th F S

I feel:
(please circle)

because _____ _____
because _____ _____
because _____ _____
because _____ _____
because _____ _____

Today I Am Grateful For

1. _____
2. _____
3. _____

What could help transform today into a remarkable day?

Reflective Writing

How has self-compassion helped me become more resilient?

_____

_____

_____

_____

_____

_____

_____

How does self-compassion differ from self-esteem?

a. Self-compassion focuses on being kind to oneself, while self-esteem is based on external validation.
b. Self-compassion involves comparing oneself to others, while self-esteem is based on self-acceptance.
c. Self-compassion
a. involves accepting one's flaws and failures, while self-esteem is based on constant self-improvement.
d. Self-compassion and self-esteem are interchangeable terms.

Answer: a. Self-compassion focuses on being kind to oneself, while self-esteem is based on external validation.

Date ___ / ___ / ___: S   M   T   W   Th   F   S

I feel:
(please circle)

because   because   because   because   because
_____   _____   _____   _____   _____
_____   _____   _____   _____   _____

Today I Am Grateful For

1. _____
2. _____
3. _____

What could help transform today into a remarkable day?

Reflective Writing

What do I need to do to become more comfortable with self-compassion?

_____

_____

_____

_____

_____

_____

_____

Which of the following is NOT a way to practice self-compassion?

a. Speaking to yourself with kindness and empathy
b. Setting unrealistic expectations and pushing oneself to achieve them
c. Engaging in self-care activities that nourish and restore you
d. Recognizing and accepting your own limitations and imperfections

Answer: b. Setting unrealistic expectations and pushing oneself to achieve them

Date ___ / ___ / ___ : S   M   T   W   Th   F   S

I feel:
(please circle)

because   because   because   because   because
_____   _____   _____   _____   _____
_____   _____   _____   _____   _____

Today I Am Grateful For

1. _____
2. _____
3. _____

What could help transform today into a remarkable day?

Reflective Writing
What are the benefits of self-compassion?

_____

_____

_____

_____

_____

_____

_____

_____

_____

What is the role of self-compassion in managing stress?

a. It increases stress levels by promoting self-acceptance.
b. It helps individuals ignore and suppress their stress.
c. It reduces stress levels by offering kindness and understanding to oneself.
d. It has no impact on stress levels.

Answer: c. It reduces stress levels by offering kindness and understanding to oneself.

Date ___ / ___ / ___ : S M T W Th F S

I feel:
(please circle)

because _____ because _____ because _____ because _____ because _____

Today I Am Grateful For

1. _____
2. _____
3. _____

What could help transform today into a remarkable day?

Reflective Writing

What are the obstacles to practicing self-compassion?

_____

_____

_____

_____

_____

_____

_____

How does self-compassion contribute to personal growth?

a. It prevents individuals from seeking self-improvement and growth.
b. It helps individuals accept their current circumstances and
a. acknowledge their strengths.
b. It promotes a constant state of self-criticism and dissatisfaction.
c. It does not have any impact on personal growth.

Answer: b. It helps individuals accept their current circumstances and acknowledge their strengths.

Date ___ / ___ / ___ : S   M   T   W   Th   F   S

I feel:
(please circle)

because   because   because   because   because

_____ _____ _____ _____ _____

_____ _____ _____ _____ _____

Today I Am Grateful For

1. _____
2. _____
3. _____

What could help transform today into a remarkable day?

Reflective Writing

What new skills have I developed through self-compassion practice?

_____

_____

_____

_____

_____

_____

_____

Which of the following is NOT a common barrier to practicing self-compassion?

a. Fear of appearing weak or self-indulgent
b. Cultural or societal norms that discourage self-care
c. Lack of self-awareness or understanding of self-compassion
d. Strong self-esteem and self-acceptance

Answer: d. Strong self-esteem and self-acceptance

Date ___ / ___ / ___ : S   M   T   W   Th   F   S

I feel:
(please circle)

because   because   because   because   because
_____ _____ _____ _____ _____
_____ _____ _____ _____ _____

Today I Am Grateful For

1. _____
2. _____
3. _____

What could help transform today into a remarkable day?

Reflective Writing

How do I use self-compassion to forgive myself?

_____

_____

_____

_____

_____

_____

_____

_____

How can mindfulness support the practice of self-compassion?

a. Mindfulness helps individuals detach from their emotions and avoid self-compassion.
b. Mindfulness allows individuals to observe their experiences without judgment, creating space for self-compassion.
c. Mindfulness increases self-criticism and prevents individuals from accepting themselves.
d. Mindfulness has no impact on self-compassion.

Answer: b. Mindfulness allows individuals to observe their experiences without judgment, creating space for self-compassion.

Date ___ / ___ / ___ : S M T W Th F S

I feel:
(please circle)

because because because because because

_____ _____ _____ _____ _____

_____ _____ _____ _____ _____

Today I Am Grateful For

1. _____
2. _____
3. _____

What could help transform today into a remarkable day?

Reflective Writing

How do I use self-compassion to move forward?

_____

_____

_____

_____

_____

_____

_____

_____

_____

How does self-compassion relate to resilience?

a. a. Self-compassion promotes a victim mentality and inhibits resilience.
b. b. Self-compassion allows individuals to bounce back from adversity and develop resilience.
c. c. Self-compassion and resilience are unrelated concepts.
d. d. Self-compassion only benefits individuals who are already resilient.

Answer: b. Self-compassion allows individuals to bounce back from adversity and develop resilience.

Date ___ / ___ / ___ : S   M   T   W   Th   F   S

I feel:
(please circle)

because   because   because   because   because
_____ _____ _____ _____ _____
_____ _____ _____ _____ _____

Today I Am Grateful For

1. _____
2. _____
3. _____

What could help transform today into a remarkable day?

Reflective Writing

What have I learned about self-care through
practicing self-compassion?

_____

_____

_____

_____

_____

_____

_____

Which of the following is a common misconception about self-compassion?

a. Self-compassion is a form of self-pity or self-indulgence.
b. Self-compassion is only relevant during times of extreme hardship.
c. Self-compassion is a sign of weakness or lack of self-discipline.
d. Self-compassion means prioritizing one's own needs above others.

Answer: d. Self-compassion means prioritizing one's own needs above others.

Date ___ / ___ / ___ : S M T W Th F S

I feel:
(please circle)

☺ because _____ _____

😁 because _____ _____

😋 because _____ _____

😣 because _____ _____

😠 because _____ _____

Today I Am Grateful For

1. _____
2. _____
3. _____

What could help transform today into a remarkable day?

Reflective Writing

How can I use self-compassion to become more mindful?

_____

_____

_____

_____

_____

_____

_____

Which of the following is an example of self-compassionate self-talk?

a. "I'm such a failure, I can never do anything right."
b. "Everyone else is so much better than me, I'll never measure up."
c. "It's okay to make mistakes, it's a part of being human."
d. "I can't believe I messed up again, I'll never be good enough.

Answer: c. "It's okay to make mistakes, it's a part of being human."

"In today's rush, we all think too much, seek too much, want too much, and forget about the joy of just being."

Eckhart Tolle

Practicing self-compassion can be a powerful tool for personal growth and transformation.

Reflective writing questions about self-compassion can help one to explore their feelings, beliefs, and experiences with self-compassion.

Questions may range from exploring the benefits of self-compassion to the obstacles to practicing self-compassion.

Other questions may focus on the skills developed through

- self-compassion practice
- how self-compassion has changed one's relationship with themselves,
- how self-compassion can help one to forgive themselves and move forward.

Practicing self-compassion can help one to become more mindful and develop a healthier relationship with themselves.

Reflective Writing

The End

As you close the pages of this mindfulness journal, remember that each word you've written is a step on your journey towards self-awareness and inner peace. Embrace the moments of clarity, the revelations, and even the uncertainties you've encountered along the way. Let this journal be a testament to your growth and a reminder that every day offers a new opportunity to be present, to observe, and to appreciate the simple wonders of life. Carry these lessons forward, and may your path be filled with mindful moments and serene reflections. Until we meet again in these pages, be gentle with yourself and stay anchored in the now.

Mindfulness isn't difficult, we just need to remember to do it.

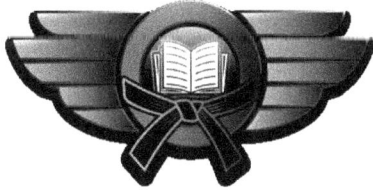

Thank You!

If you found this book helpful, I would be grateful if you would **post an honest review on Amazon** so this book can reach other supportive readers like you!

All you need to do is digitally flip to the back and leave your review. Or visit amazon.com/author/senseipauldavid click the correct book cover and click on the blue link next to the yellow stars that say, "customer reviews."

As always...
It's a great day to be alive!

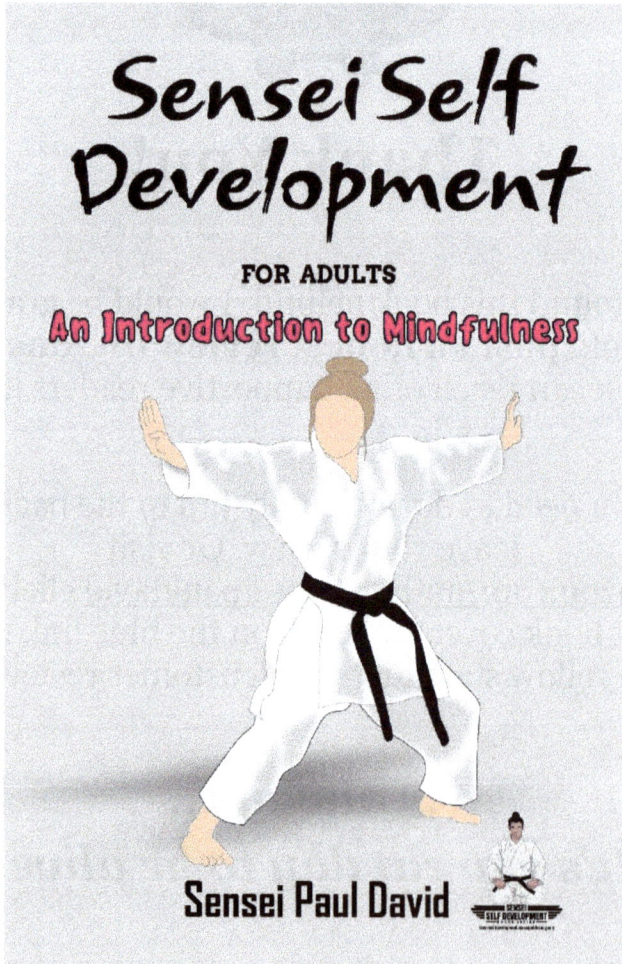

Sensei Self Development

FOR ADULTS

An Introduction to Mindfulness

Sensei Paul David

Check Out The SSD Chronicles
Series CLICK HERE

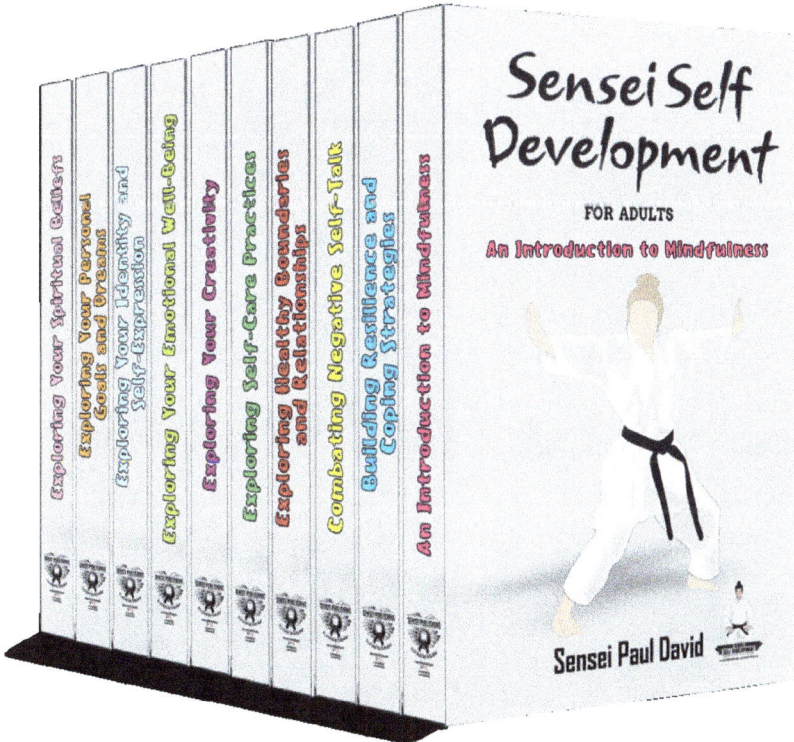

Get/Share Your FREE All-Ages Mental Health eBook Now at

www.senseiselfdevelopment.com

Or CLICK HERE

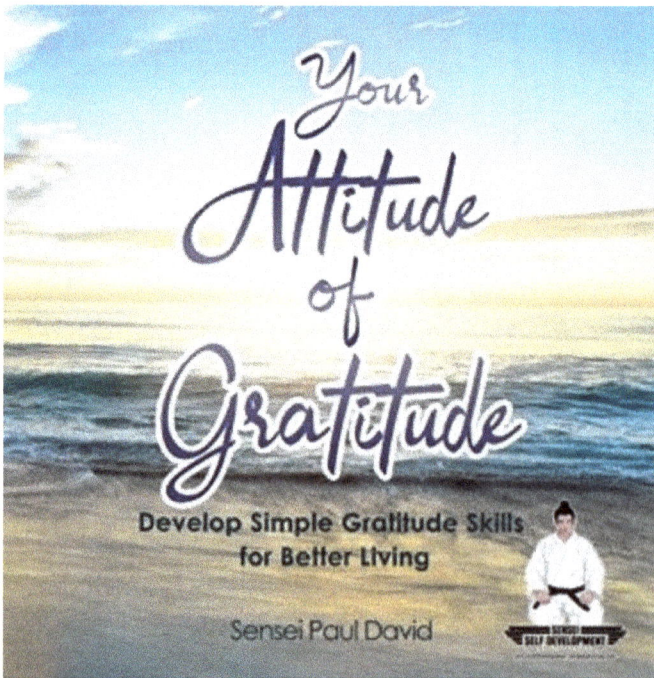

senseiselfdevelopment.com

Click Another Book In The SSD BOOK SERIES:

senseipublishing.com/SSD_SERIES

CLICK HERE

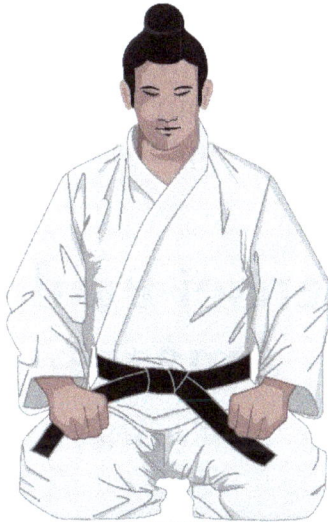

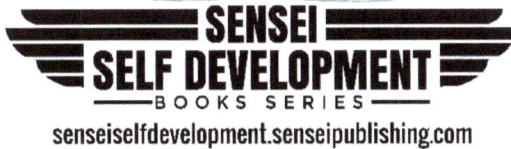

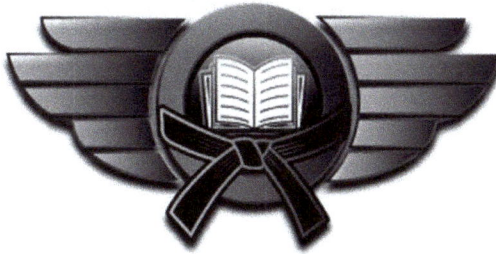

Join Our Publishing Journey!

If you would like to receive FREE BOOKS, please visit **www.senseipublishing.com**. Join our newsletter by entering your email address in the pop-up box

Follow Sensei Paul David on Amazon

CLICK THE LOGO BELOW

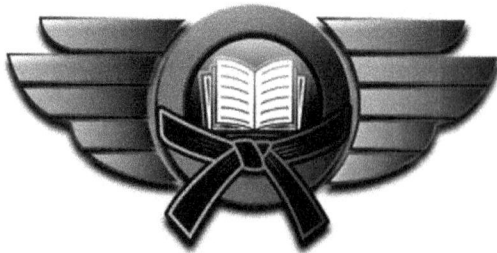

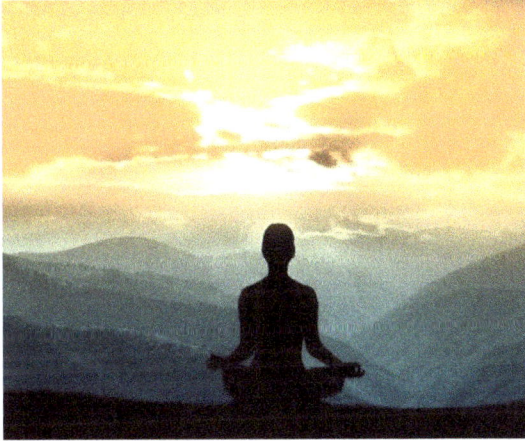

FREE BONUS!!!
Experience Over 25 FREE Engaging Guided Meditations!

Prized Skills & Practices for Adults & Kids. Help Restore Deep-Sleep, Lower Stress, Improve Posture, Navigate Uncertainty & More.

Download the Free Insight Timer App and click the link below:
http://insig.ht/sensei_paul

About Sensei Publishing

Sensei Publishing commits itself to helping people of all ages transform into better versions of themselves by providing high-quality and research-based self-development books with an emphasis on mental health and guided meditations. Sensei Publishing offers well-written e-books, audiobooks, paperbacks and online courses that simplify complicated but practical topics in line with its mission to inspire people towards positive transformation.

It's a great day to be alive!

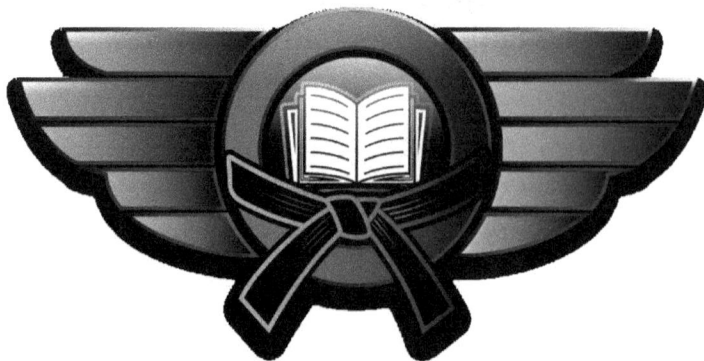

About the Author

I create simple & transformative eBooks & Guided Meditations for Adults & Children proven to help navigate uncertainty, solve niche problems & bring families closer together.

I'm a former finance project manager, private pilot, jiu-jitsu instructor, musician & former University of Toronto Fitness Trainer. I prefer a science-based approach to focus on these & other areas in my life to stay humble & hungry to evolve. I hope you enjoy my work and I'd love to hear your feedback.

- It's a great day to be alive!

Sensei Paul David

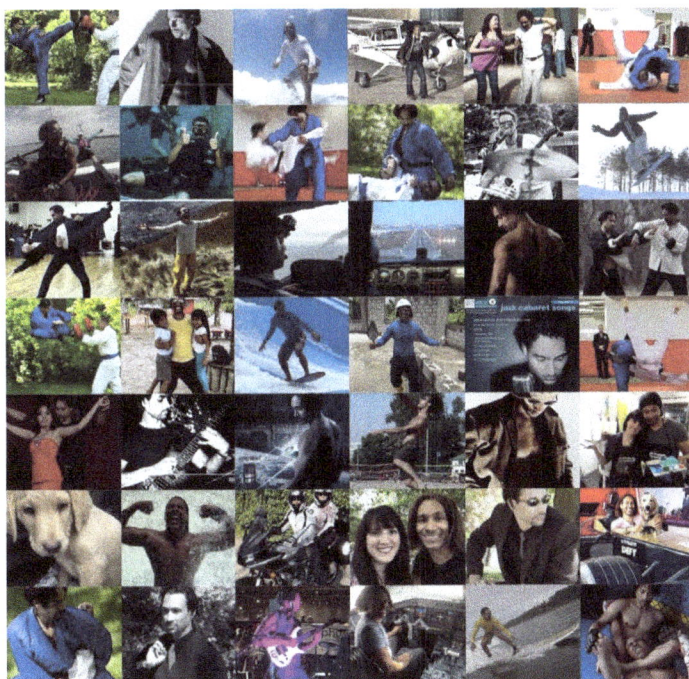

Scan & Follow/Like/Subscribe: Facebook, Instagram,
YouTube: @senseipublishing

Scan using your phone/iPad camera for Social Media
Visit us at www.senseipublishing.com and sign up for our
newsletter to learn more about our exciting books and to
experience our FREE Guided Meditations for Kids & Adults.

www.ingramcontent.com/pod-product-compliance
Lightning Source LLC
Chambersburg PA
CBHW071243020426
42333CB00015B/1609